WALTER BISHOP

Cool Your Body, Calm Your Mind

Explore the Benefits of Cold Water Therapy for Improved Grit, Sleep, Recovery, and More Energy with Reduced Stress

This book was professionally typeset on Reedsy.
Find out more at reedsy.com

Contents

I

Part One

1

Introduction

Are you feeling exhausted even after a full night's rest? Do you struggle with stress and anxiety in your daily life? If so, "Cool Your Body, Calm Your Mind" is the book for you! This guide to Cold Water Therapy will provide you with evidence-based knowledge to improve your well-being. The therapy is accessible to anyone and can help you meet the demands of daily life. Through each chapter, you will learn about the science behind this powerful tool and its benefits. Discover how Cold Water Therapy can help you:

- Reduce stress.
- Promote better sleep.
- Increase energy
- Preventing neurodegenerative
- Building Resilience
- Recover faster

With practical tips and information, you can easily incorporate this method into your daily routine and change your mindset. Join the ranks of high-performing individuals who have already found success with Cold Water Therapy. Take charge of your health and well-being today by reading "Cool Your Body, Calm Your Mind".

In the book, the term Cold Water Therapy (CWT) is used synonymously with Cold Water Immersion (CWI) and cold hydrotherapy. When differences arise, the book goes into more detail about these differences.

2

The Science of Cold Water Therapy

Have you heard about the growing trend of CWT and its associated health benefits? But what exactly is cold water therapy, and what does the science say about its benefits?

CWT, also known as cold hydrotherapy, involves the use of water at around 59°F (15°C) to stimulate health benefits or treat health conditions. This practice has been around for centuries, with recent adaptations including ice baths, outdoor swims, and cold water immersion therapy sessions. CWI is a specific type of cold water therapy that can improve the body's natural recovery process. Taking ice baths or cold showers on a regular basis can activate the body's natural healing powers, reduce muscle inflammation, improve cardiovascular circulation, facilitate weight loss and much more.

In this book, we'll explore the science behind CWT and provide insights into the benefits and safety considerations of this practice. So, if you're curious about the positive effects of CWT, read on to learn more!

2:1 The Physiological Benefits of Cold Water Therapy

Hydrotherapy is the use of water to treat various conditions. Superficial cold application can cause physiological reactions with many benefits. Just by regular winter swimming or cold showers you can achieve great health benefits, such as:

- Decrease in local metabolic function
- Local edema
- Nerve conduction velocity
- Muscle spasm
- Increase in local anesthetic effects.
- Decreased tension
- Fatigue
- Memory and mood negative state points improved general well-being.
- Pain relief for those who suffer from rheumatism, fibromyalgia and asthma.

One hour head-out water immersions at different temperatures (32°C, 20°C, and 14°C) produced various effects. Immersion at 32°C lowered the heart rate, blood pressure, plasma renin activity, plasma cortisol, and aldosterone concentrations, and increased diuresis. Immersion at 20°C produced similar effects but with increased metabolic rate. Immersion at 14°C lowered temperature and increased metabolic rate, heart rate, blood pressure, plasma noradrenaline and dopamine concentrations, and diuresis, with increased plasma aldosterone concentration. However, hormone production was not related to changes in temperature.

2.2 How Cold Water Therapy Affects the Nervous system.

The nervous system plays a significant role in the therapeutic effects of various modalities such as cold water immersion, aquatic therapy, sauna bath, and colon cleansing. These modalities have been shown to affect nerve conduction, activate parasympathetic or sympathetic nerve activity, and stimulate various components of the central nervous system.

For example, cold modalities such as ice massage, ice pack, and CWI have been found to reduce skin temperature and sensory nerve conduction, with CWI being the most effective modality for reducing motor nerve conduction. Aquatic therapy, on the other hand, can block nociceptors by acting on thermal receptors and mechanoreceptors, leading to positive effects on spinal segmental mechanisms.

Sauna bath has been shown to increase heart rate during the sauna phase and decrease diastolic blood pressure during the postsauna phase in paraplegic and tetraplegic groups. Colon cleansing has also been found to significantly improve the mental state of individuals with schizophrenia, who often experience co-morbid intestinal illnesses.

Overall, these modalities can have a significant impact on the nervous system and may provide therapeutic benefits for various conditions such as multiple sclerosis, Parkinson's disease, and chronic pain.

3

How Cold Water Therapy Reduces Stress

Have you ever heard of cold showers being used as a natural remedy for muscle aches or to wake you up quickly in the morning? What you may not know is that cold showers can also potentially help manage anxiety symptoms when used as water therapy or hydrotherapy.

Anxiety is a common mental health condition that causes excessive fear and worry. While it's normal to experience occasional anxiety and stress, anxiety disorders can interfere with your daily activities and make it difficult to participate in work and social activities. Although there are many different ways to treat chronic anxiety, some complementary therapies like cold showers may be worth exploring.

Before you rush into a cold shower, it's important to consider whether braving colder water will actually help alleviate your anxiety symptoms. It's also important to talk to your doctor about other ways to manage anxiety for the long term.

While there's still more research needed to prove that cold showers are an effective treatment for anxiety, some studies suggest that hydrotherapy may have similar benefits for anxiety management. For example, a 2008 study found that hydrotherapy helped improve symptoms of depression in participants who took 2- to 3-minute cold water showers at 68°F (20°C), one to two times per day.

Cold showers have also been proven to help improve blood circulation and increase endorphins, or the feel-good hormones in your brain. Additionally, cold water may decrease cortisol, a stress-inducing hormone. For athletes, ice baths are commonly used to decrease inflammation that may lead to muscle soreness after an intense workout. Similarly, a cold shower may help manage inflammation associated with anxiety.

Using hydrotherapy for anxiety requires using cold water for only a few minutes at a time, followed by a warm or lukewarm shower. Additionally, focusing on the sensation of the cold water can temporarily take your mind off of the things that may be causing your anxiety, helping you stay present in the moment.

In conclusion, while more research is needed to fully understand the effectiveness of cold showers as an anxiety treatment, there are promising signs that hydrotherapy may help alleviate some symptoms. As with any complementary therapy, it's important to talk to your doctor before trying cold showers for anxiety management.

4

Building Resilience & Grit!

Grit is about having a strong and persistent character, an ability to stick to goals and persevere through challenges. Cold exposure can be a powerful tool for developing grit because it requires individuals to face discomfort and stress in a deliberate and controlled way. When you deliberately expose yourself to cold temperatures, you are intentionally putting yourself in a stressful situation that requires mental toughness and resilience. By repeatedly subjecting yourself to this stressor and learning to manage your physical and emotional responses, you can develop greater mental fortitude and a stronger sense of grit.

This is because the process of deliberately exposing yourself to stressors and practicing top-down control, as discussed earlier, helps build neural pathways in the brain that support resilience and grit. By learning to exert control over your body's automatic responses, you can build a greater sense of agency and control over your own life, which is a hallmark of grit. When you subject yourself to the cold, you're not just toughening up your body - you're also building mental fortitude. By intentionally exposing yourself to a stressor, you're taking control of your body's reflexive responses and exerting what's known as 'top-down control'. This process involves your prefrontal cortex - the area of your brain responsible for planning and suppressing impulsivity.

But the benefits of deliberate cold exposure don't end there. This top-down control process is the foundation of resilience and grit, allowing you to face any challenge with a calm and clear mind. As you train your mind to handle the stress of the cold, you're also building the skills you need to cope with real-world stressors outside of the icy environment. So don't shy away from the challenge of cold exposure - embrace it as an opportunity to become the best version of yourself. With each exposure, you're building mental strength and resilience that will serve you for a lifetime. Start training your mind today and see what incredible feats you're capable of achieving!

5

How cold water therapy improves sleep

Taking a cold shower or spending time in a cold plunge is a form of cold therapy that has gained popularity in recent years due to its many health benefits. Some of the benefits include improved circulation, decreased inflammation, reduced muscle soreness, and increased energy. However, one aspect of cold therapy that is often overlooked is its impact on sleep quality.

When you take a cold shower or spend time in a cold plunge, your body's temperature will decrease dramatically. This drop in temperature causes your body to release chemicals such as melatonin, which researchers believe induces sleep. Melatonin is a hormone that is naturally produced by the body to regulate sleep-wake cycles. It helps to signal to the brain that it is time to sleep and plays a crucial role in our ability to fall asleep and stay asleep throughout the night.

However, cold therapy can also cause a spike in cortisol levels, which is also known as the stress hormone. Cortisol is a chemical that the body produces in response to stress. While cortisol is necessary for our bodies to function properly, high levels of cortisol at night can lead to poor sleep quality. Research has shown that increased cortisol levels at night are associated with difficulty falling asleep, difficulty staying asleep, and non-restorative sleep.

Therefore, timing is crucial when it comes to CWT and its impact on sleep quality. It's best to time your cold plunge or shower 1-2 hours before bed to allow your body time to respond to the new stimulus and reach the ideal core temperature for sleep. It's important to note that cold therapy before bed may not be relaxing. Feeling your body warm up after a cold shower can create feelings of relaxation, but the initial cold can be highly stressful if you're not used to it. Therefore, it's important to consider the timing of your cold therapy before bed and condition yourself to cold water gradually.

That's why many people prefer to take cold showers or a cold plunge in the morning or early afternoon. By taking a cold plunge or shower, you can jump-start your day and feel more alert and focused, which then leads to better sleep. Performing CWI early in the day is an important aspect of cold therapy that is often overlooked. In the next chapter, we will discuss the importance of time and the benefits of performing the intervention early in the day from a different point of view.

6

Enhancing Energy and Neurogenesis through Cold Water Therapy.

C WT has been shown to have numerous benefits for the brain, including increasing levels of norepinephrine and dopamine. These effects occur due to the top-down control process that takes place when individuals embrace the stress of cold exposure as a challenge, involving the prefrontal cortex. This process develops resilience and grit, which can be applied in real-life situations outside of the cold environment.

Cold exposure also protects against neurodegenerative diseases and traumatic brain injuries. Exposure to the cold triggers the release of RNA binding motif 3 (RBM3), which promotes the regeneration of synapses in the brain, preventing cognitive decline. RBM3 plays a crucial role in neuroplasticity, repairing and regenerating synapses, and is found in the brain, heart, liver, and skeletal muscle.

Cold exposure significantly increases norepinephrine levels, up to 500%, and this hormone is involved in stress responses, attention, and focus. The increased levels of norepinephrine have been linked to neurogenesis, which is the process of producing neurons by neural stem cells. CWT is a potential protective therapy that can help improve cognitive deficits caused by traumatic brain injury.

Dopamine is essential for our cognitive and physical well-being, playing a role in executive function, motor control, motivation, reinforcement, and reward. Dopamine disorders can lead to a decline in these key functions, affecting our ability to learn and thrive. In particular, Parkinson's disease, which is the second most common neurodegenerative disorder, is associated with the loss of dopaminergic neurons in the substantia nigra pars compacta (SNc).

Interestingly, CWT has been found to activate the release of dopamine in addition to norepinephrine. This is why people who undergo CWT often feel incredible afterward. Furthermore, cold water therapy shows promise in the treatment of neurodegenerative diseases like Alzheimer's and Parkinson's.

In summary, dopamine plays a crucial role in our cognitive and physical health, and any disruption in its function can have severe consequences. Fortunately, innovative treatments like CWT can activate the release of dopamine and may help in preventing or treating neurodegenerative diseases. Cold exposure also triggers the release of RBM3, promoting the regeneration of synapses and preventing cognitive decline. Cold water therapy is a potential protective therapy that can improve cognitive deficits caused by traumatic brain injury.

7

Recover faster.

Cold water therapy, also known as cold-water immersion or ice baths, is a recovery method that is becoming increasingly popular among athletes. A meta-analysis of cold-water immersion effects on recovery found that it can be highly effective after high-intensity exercise or endurance training. In particular, short interval (< 5 mins) cold water immersion has demonstrated positive outcomes for muscle power, perceived recovery, and decreased muscle soreness. This is partly due to a reduction in circulating creatine kinases.

However, it is important to note that CWI can limit some of the gains in hypertrophy, strength, or endurance if done in the 4 hours after training. To avoid this, it is better to wait 6 to 8 or more hours until after training, or do it before training. Unless your goal is simply to recover without adaptation, such as when in competition mode and not trying to get better, stronger, etc.

But what is the science behind these claims? Many experts in exercise physiology have studied the effects of cold water therapy on muscle recovery and performance. Cooling can reduce nerve impulse transmission and induce constriction of blood vessels in peripheral tissues, which results in reduced fluid diffusion that may assist in reducing exercise-induced acute inflammation. This is effective at reducing the symptoms of exercise-induced delayed onset muscle soreness.

Additionally, ice baths can influence our minds as well as our muscles. A research study compared the effects of an ice bath with a placebo condition that participants were tricked into thinking was as effective as an ice bath. The results showed that participants in both conditions rated their belief in the benefits of their assigned recovery condition similarly, which translated into similar recovery of leg extension strength over a 48-hour post-exercise period.

Although ice baths can help muscles recover, it may follow that they can improve sports performance. However, it is not that simple as scientific studies show varying outcomes regarding the effect of post-exercise ice baths on subsequent performance. The effects of ice baths on exercise performance differ depending on what kind of exercise is involved. For example, after strength exercise, CWI may actually hinder the benefits of exercise. It can lead to reductions and/or blunting of the desired results from strength training, such as increasing strength and muscle mass, and cellular improvements within the muscle.

On the other hand, the effects on endurance training may be quite different. Cooling the exercised muscle increases the cellular signal which turns on mitochondrial biogenesis, which is one of the positive effects that comes from endurance training. Therefore, ice baths could help to amplify this benefit.

In summary, cold water therapy can be a highly effective recovery tool after high-intensity exercise or endurance training. However, it is important to use caution when using it after strength training. Instead, its use following one-off circumstances like big sports events or endurance exercise is recommended, and may even provide additional benefits for subsequent endurance exercise performance.

8

Incorporate Cold Water Therapy into Your Life.

Starting the day off with physical exercise can be a game-changer. Whether it's swimming, weight lifting, or jogging, getting your blood pumping and your body moving can set you up for a productive and energized day ahead.

After your workout, it's time to incorporate cold water therapy into your daily routine. The practice has numerous benefits, such as delaying cognitive decline and Alzheimer's disease, and some of the effects are immediate, like a surge of dopamine and increased energy levels.

But, it's essential to take necessary precautions when engaging in CWT. If you're new to the practice, start with shorter exposures and gradually work your way up. With consistency, you can build up your tolerance and progress from cold showers to ice baths.

When performing cold water therapy, it's important to keep in mind that the purpose of the exercise can influence when you perform it to maximize its benefits. Whether you're looking to reduce inflammation, improve circulation, or boost your immune system, the timing of your CWI can make a significant difference in the outcomes you experience.

Don't let the fear of cold water stop you from experiencing the incredible benefits of this practice. Embrace the challenge and push yourself to new limits. With patience, perseverance, and a willingness to step out of your comfort zone. With the right tools, you may be amazed at the transformative effects it can have on your mind, body, and spirit.

7.1 Precautions and advice on cold water therapy before starting

The act of immersing yourself in cold water can have significant effects on your body. Cold water immersion can cause changes in your blood pressure, heart rate, and circulation, which can lead to serious cardiac stress. This stress can be severe enough to cause heart attacks, which can result in death. Unfortunately, there have been documented cases of both cold exposure and heart attacks occurring during open water swim events.

Therefore, it is important to discuss the potential risks of cold water immersion with your doctor to determine if it is safe for you to try. Your doctor can assess your overall health and advise you on any precautions you should take before attempting CWI. It's always better to be cautious and well-informed when it comes to your health, so don't hesitate to seek professional advice before taking the plunge.

When you're ready to take the plunge and try it out for yourself, here are some suggestions to get started:

- One suggestion is to take warm-to-cold showers, starting with warm water and gradually decreasing the temperature after a few minutes. Alternatively, skipping the warmup and jumping straight into a cold shower may be especially beneficial after exercise.

- Another option is to immerse oneself in an ice bath, adding ice to water until the temperature reaches between 10°C and 15°C (50°F and 59°F), and staying submerged for only 10 to 15 minutes.

- Finally, considering a short swim in colder waters is also suggested as a way to expose oneself to cold temperatures. It is important to keep in mind that these methods of cold exposure may not be suitable for everyone, and it is recommended to consult with a healthcare professional before starting any new cold exposure regimen.

Here is some advice on how to push yourself. When exposing yourself to cold temperatures, you may experience mental resistance in the form of internal dialogue telling you not to do it. This mental resistance can be thought of as "walls" that need to be overcome. These walls are actually caused by adrenaline in your brain and body, which is what triggers the adaptive response that leads to physical and mental changes. If overcoming the challenge of cold exposure were easy, then there would be no stimulus for your body to change and adapt. Therefore, it is essential to maintain control over your reflexive urge to leave the cold environment. One way to do this is by counting the walls and setting a goal to traverse a certain number of them during each round of exposure (for example, 3-5 walls). Alternatively, you could set a time goal. Using the walls approach has several advantages. It can help you to overcome mental barriers and develop a stronger mind-body connection. Additionally, it can be applied to other stressful situations in life, as most stressors do not have a clear endpoint that can be timed. Overall, the walls approach can help you to overcome mental resistance and develop greater resilience in the face of challenges.

9

Conclusion

Cold water therapy involves exposing yourself to cold water in various forms, such as cold showers or ice baths, for therapeutic benefits. While many may shy away from the idea of voluntarily submerging themselves in cold water, the potential benefits may be worth considering.

One benefit of cold water therapy is its potential to reduce stress. Cold water exposure has been shown to activate the sympathetic nervous system and increase the production of noradrenaline, a hormone that can help reduce stress and anxiety. In addition, the shock of the cold water can shift your focus away from stressors and help you develop resilience to stress over time.

Another potential benefit is better recovery. Cold water therapy has been shown to decrease inflammation, which can help speed up recovery after exercise or injury. Athletes have long used ice baths to help reduce muscle soreness and speed up recovery time after intense workouts.

Improving sleep is also a potential benefit of cold water therapy.

Exposure to cold water has been shown to increase the production of melatonin, a hormone that helps regulate sleep. Additionally, the increase in noradrenaline production may help improve overall sleep quality.

Cold water therapy may also help improve GRIT, or the ability to persevere through challenges. By exposing yourself to cold water regularly, you can develop mental toughness and resilience that can carry over to other areas of your life.

Increased energy levels are another potential benefit of cold water therapy. The shock of the cold water can help increase alertness and wakefulness, while the increase in noradrenaline production can also provide a boost of energy.

Finally, cold water therapy may help promote neurogenesis, or the growth of new neurons in the brain. This may lead to improved cognitive function and a decreased risk of age-related cognitive decline.

Incorporating cold water therapy into your daily routine may seem daunting, but starting small can help. Begin with ending your shower with a blast of cold water for a few seconds, then gradually increase the time and intensity of the cold exposure. Additionally, using a pool or ice bath can be an effective way to experience the benefits of CWT. Remember to always listen to your body and consult with a medical professional if you have any concerns.

In conclusion, while the idea of voluntarily exposing yourself to cold water may seem uncomfortable, the potential benefits of CWI are numerous. From reducing stress to improving cognitive function, incorporating CWT into your routine may be worth considering for a healthier, happier you.

10

Elevating Body and Mind!

I am delighted that you have chosen to explore my insights and experiences. This book contains valuable tools and advice that will help you achieve your goals and unlock your full potential. But why stop there? By following the QR code to my social media page, you can discover even more of my work and my books. You'll get exclusive insights into my latest projects and the opportunity to interact with me and like-minded individuals. You can also take a look at my additional book, "Defending The Aging Brain", which offers insights into maintaining brain health and fighting against cognitive decline.

I am confident that this book will be of great help to you, and I invite you to follow my social media page to continue your journey towards personal and professional development. If you have found this book useful, please feel free to share it with others.

Thank you for choosing to read my book, and I look forward to sharing more knowledge and inspiration with you on my social media page.

11

Resources

Stanborough, R. M. J. (2020, July 8). *What to Know About Cold Water Therapy*. Healthline. https://www.healthline.com/health/cold-water-therapy

Wim Hof Method. (n.d.). *Wim Hof Method - Join Our New Platform.* https://www.wimhofmethod.com/cold-water-therapy

Mooventhan, A. (2014, May 1). *Scientific evidence-based effects of hydrotherapy on various systems of the body Mooventhan A, Nivethitha L - North Am J Med Sci.* https://www.najms.org/article.asp?issn=1947-2714;year=2014;volume=6;issue=5;spage=199;epage=209;aulast=Mooventhan

Cherney, K. (2020, June 22). *Cold Shower for Anxiety: Does It Help?* Healthline. https://www.healthline.com/health/anxiety/cold-shower-for-anxiety

Huberman, A. (2023, February 9). *The Science & Use of Cold Exposure for Health & Performance*. Huberman Lab. https://hubermanlab.com/the-science-and-use-of-cold-exposure-for-health-and-performance/

JumpX Marketing. (2022, February 9). *Cold Therapy Before Bed For Improved Sleep?* PLUNGE. https://thecoldplunge.com/blogs/blog/cold-therapy-before-bed-sleep

Nall, R. M. (2021, April 7). *How a Cold Shower Before Bed Affects Your Sleep.* Healthline. https://www.healthline.com/health/how-a-cold-shower-before-bed-affects-your-sleep

Fullerton, L. (2022, June 24). *Neuroprotection and neuroplasticity benefits of cold water therapy.* Monk. https://discovermonk.com/blogs/blog/neuroprotection-and-neuroplasticity-benefits-of-cold-water-therapy

M. (2021, September 26). *Do Ice Baths Actually Improve Muscle Recovery? Read This Before You Try It Out:* ScienceAlert. https://www.sciencealert.com/do-ice-baths-actually-improve-muscle-recovery-read-this-before-you-try

Stanborough, R. M. J. (2020b, July 8). *What to Know About Cold Water Therapy.* Healthline. https://www.healthline.com/health/cold-water-therapy